Revalidation for nurses and midwives

CLAUDIA TOMLINSON

Copyright © 2016 Claudia Tomlinson

All rights reserved.

ISBN-10: 1519209754
ISBN-13: 978-1519209757

CONTENTS

1	Introduction	Pg. 1
2	Planning your revalidation journey	Pg. 11
3	Practice Hours	Pg. 15
4	Continuing Professional Development	Pg. 19
5	Practice-related feedback and reflective accounts	Pg. 24
6	Reflective discussion and confirmation	Pg. 31
7	Application and verification	Pg. 47
8	Revalidation in diverse settings	Pg. 50
9	Social media and revalidation	Pg. 60
10	Lessons learned so far	Pg. 68
	References and resources	Pg. 73
	About the author	Pg. 74

1 INTRODUCTION

Since April 2016, nurses and midwives registered by the Nursing and Midwifery Council (NMC) have been renewing their registration through the new revalidation process. Following the processing of the first cohort of revalidation applicants, the NMC hailed the process 'a major success' (NMC May, 2016). The NMC has published the first quarterly report on revalidation available in August 2016. It concluded:

"The data highlights that renewal rates are in line with those seen in previous years, with no evidence of revalidation having an adverse effect on the register. Across the four UK countries revalidation rates are very similar, ranging from 91 percent to 94 percent" (NMC, August 2016).

Prior to the introduction of revalidation for nurses and midwives there was some concern and anxiety about the introduction of this new system. There was concern that registrants would not receive sufficient employer support, that there would be limited access to training and development opportunities, and that those not in traditional NHS roles may particularly experience difficulties.

Revalidation is the process of formal ratification by the NMC that registrants have successfully met all of the requirements of the revalidation process and are approved for registered practice for the next three-year period. Nurses and midwives must in future renew their registration through the new revalidation process. Failure to revalidate, by not meeting the new requirements, means that nurses and midwives' registrations will lapse and they will automatically stop being able to practice as a nurse or midwife in England, Wales, Scotland and Northern Ireland. They will then need to re-apply to the NMC to re-join the register.

Registrants will continue to pay an annual retention fee to maintain their registration with the NMC, and every three years will go through a renewal process. Revalidation has now replaced its predecessor, PREP.

PREP (Post-Registration Education and Practice) was the regulatory framework for the renewal of NMC registrations and is no longer effective. Revalidation builds on and enhances the PREP framework. The PREP framework had a Practice Standard of a minimum number of practice hours requirement over three years, and a CPD standard of a minimum of 35 hours learning activity over the same period.

On renewal, registrants were required to complete a Notification of Practice form upon which they need to declare they have met the standards, and that they are of good health and character. One of the main reasons PREP was considered to be not fit for the purpose of maintaining professional standards was that it was an entirely self-validating with no third party check before renewal. PREP included a process by which the NMC audited a sample of PREP portfolios to evaluate submissions, but the number is relatively small and most registrants have never had an independent check on their compliance with nursing standards.

A second key driver for the introduction of revalidation by the NMC is to increase registrant's engagement with the NMC Code. Under the PREP system, the Code was not well known or understood, and registrants did not have incentives to incorporate in their day to day practice. The new process of NMC revalidation is intended to weave the Code into the heart of the day to day practice of registrants.

The introduction of NMC revalidation has also brought Fitness to Practice (FTP) into sharper focus. FTP is an existing part of the NMC regulatory framework. According to the NMC, "Being fit to practice requires a nurse or midwife to have the skills, knowledge, good health and good character to do their job safely and effectively".

The NMC has powers of investigation if an allegation is made against a registrant to the effect that they do not meet the NMC standards for skills, education and behaviour. The NMC can investigate allegations of misconduct, lack of competence, criminal behaviour and serious ill health. It is important that all involved in supporting registrants with revalidation understand and are able to distinguish the difference between the two processes. The two processes are separate and the NMC intends that they remain independent processes.

Why was revalidation introduced?

In 2013, Sir Robert Francis published his report into failings in care at Mid Staffordshire:

NHS Foundation Trust Public Inquiry and made the following recommendation in relation to nurses and midwives:

"The NMC should introduce a system of revalidation similar to that of the GMC as a means of reinforcing the status and competence of registered nurses as well as providing additional protection to the public. It is essential that the NMC has the resources and the administrative and leadership skills to ensure that this does not detract from its existing core function of regulating fitness to practice." (Report of the Mid Staffordshire NHS Foundation Trust Public Inquiry, 2013)

The introduction of NMC revalidation is the response to this recommendation, intended to protect the public and improve standards of care. The NMC stated that:

"The introduction of revalidation is the most significant change to regulation in a generation and we firmly believe that it will give the public confidence that the people who care for them are continuously striving to improve their practice."

How to approach revalidation?

Revalidation should be approached in line with the guidance from the NMC as it is the only body authorised to revalidate nurses and midwives, and sets the standards and framework for the regulation of registrants. It should be approached as an opportunity to undertake professional development activities that contribute to the improvement of registrants in a meaningful way. There is a risk that in seeking to meet the new standards, registrants may lose sight of the underpinning purpose of revalidation. There is a risk that meeting the seven requirements, and successfully submitting a revalidation application is seen as the purpose of the exercise. It is in danger of being seen and treated as a 'tick-box' exercise, or another set of hoops put up for under pressure nurses and midwives to jump through. Taken as a planned, continuous cycle of professional development, registrants will experience the revalidation process as enjoyable, empowering, and a process that enhances their value in the workplace. If viewed revalidation as an ongoing process, this will ensure integrity is brought to the process and remains there throughout.

Too many nurses and midwives feel they get slim pickings in terms of CPD learning and development opportunities compared to other professional healthcare colleagues. Too many feel they are expected to be the backbone of health service provision with insufficient time and resources for them to undertake developmental activities needed to maintain standards. NMC revalidation could also bring more equitable access to CPD among nurses and midwives, as some registrants experience unequal access to CPD compared to NMC colleagues.

A final clear benefit of NMC revalidation to registrants is the opportunity for increased support and networking among nurses and midwives. Registrants will be able to organise and collaborate, and work together to support each other through the process. The benefits of NMC revalidation to employers are clear.

Peter Senge in his book The Fifth Discipline (1990), wrote about the importance of team learning in the development of a Learning Organisation, vital for organisational growth and development. In the era of highly constrained health and social care budgets, organisations are increasingly reliant on creative, innovative, flexible staff with vision and commitment to learning about new ways of working. The NMC revalidation process supports nurses and midwives to learn, improve and share learning with colleagues in the MDT, and even across organisational boundaries through the setting up of networks.

Equality and NMC revalidation

Employed registrants who will be relying on their employers to support them to meet the revalidation requirements will have expectations that this will be provided equitably to all employees who require the same support. Some employers are providing dedicated support by ring-fencing time within existing posts, or recruiting new roles specifically to look introduce and run schemes. Due to the fact that revalidation is designed on the assumption of discretionary effort and support from employers, other registrants and other staff, resources may be limited initially. Over time, employers will be able to consider increasing resources for NMC revalidation, through making the provision of support to

NMC registrants a mandatory part of job descriptions. In the interim, careful oversight and monitoring will be needed to ensure equity of access to NMC revalidation.

Employers and revalidation

The introduction of revalidation for nurses and midwives presents significant benefits for employers. Change may also inevitably bring some risks and unintended consequences. There may initially be an increase in the number of Fitness to Practice referrals by employers to the NMC as closer scrutiny is brought to bear on the work of registrants, perhaps by others with little or no prior experience of doing so. It will of course be distressing for any individual registrant that inappropriately faces FTP proceedings, however patient safety and adherence to the Code by registrants are paramount. Good employer engagement with NMC revalidation will reduce the risk of increased FTP proceedings.

There may be avoidable wastage of registrants who are taken off the register, due to lack of employer support to meet the revalidation requirements. There may be an impact on staffing levels as registrants will not be able to work as nurses and midwives if they fail to revalidate successfully. Employers will need to have a process in place for this situation, and it will probably mirror the situation where a nurse or midwife inadvertently lets their registration lapse. Nonetheless, employers may be faced with scenarios of having to employ temporary staff to cover gaps in staffing levels due to revalidation. This situation is recoverable, as registrants will be able to apply to the NMC for re-admission to the register. Employers may also face an increase in employment disputes from registrants in relation to revalidation, and this may result in staff disengagement.

Trade unions and professional bodies can provide a supportive role for employers to circumvent the potential increase for employee relations matters. Many employers are already putting strategies in place to manage these unintended consequences of NMC revalidation. Developing an organisational policy, an organisational revalidation scheme, and an a pilot for the first cohort of registrants to revalidate will provide a baseline and strong foundation from which to grow. Many organisations are identifying or appointing an NMC revalidation lead, and giving consideration to developing databases of reflective discussion partners, confirmers, and a process for nurses and midwives to access the database.

Where an employer becomes known for providing an excellent revalidation support schemes for registrants, this can serve as a pull factor in attracting and retaining nurses and midwives. Locally, employers can give consideration to including open access to free CPD events for registrants living locally, and to provide opportunities share underused IT suites by providing evening access to professional networks. These actions will contribute to the positive employer's reputation for local engagement, and for taking proactive steps for the good of the broader health and social care economy.

Why has this book been written?

This book has not been written to replace or substitute for the expert and authoritative information provided by the

NMC, but to complement what is available.

The book is based on the author's experience of preparing registrants for the process of making their online revalidation applications. In the period since the start of the new system in April 2016, the author has assisted registrants for each monthly cohort through the provision of advice, and acting as a reflective discussion partner and confirmer. The overwhelming feedback to date is that the process and experience has been much more straightforward than anticipated. This book has been written to help demystify the process. The NMC has developed a new revalidation microsite (small website area) on its main website. It is continuously updating and improving the website, with new templates, guides and new ways of presenting the information. This website is an excellent form of information

This book has primarily been written for nurses and midwives to support them through the revalidation process. There is no requirement for registrants to acquire additional resources to the guidance provided by the NMC on the revalidation pages of its website. The NMC has published a comprehensive set of guidance documents, worked examples, and resources that will enable registrants to complete the process. This book is not intended as alternative reading or a substitute for reviewing the guidance. It is essential that all registrants seeking to revalidate satisfies themselves of the guidance and mandatory elements as set out by the NMC.

This book is for those who wish to have a book to complement other published materials, and to support their wider thinking about NMC revalidation. It provides an opportunity to explore and consider a range of contextual, organisational, cultural and professional factors to reflect on during the process. The NMC focuses their guidance on the compliance and regulatory requirements, and this book enhances that through the provision of more detailed opportunity to think through the issues and implications of

revalidation.

This book provides an overview of some of the challenges that some registrants in diverse settings and scopes of practice may face, and suggestions for overcoming these. This book has also been written to raise the profile of NMC revalidation. The book may also be useful for employers, who want a broader context and consideration of the issues of NMC revalidation.

The book may be of interest to those involved in organisational quality, transformation, and patient experience. Those acting in the role of line managers and confirmers, particularly those unfamiliar with NMC regulation may find the book useful for providing background and context. Patients, carers and those who use services provided by registrants, and the general reader may be interested to read about the changes and contribute to opportunities to comment on, and discuss the impact of NMC revalidation on their experience of the quality of care, which is the purpose of its introduction.

2 PLANNING YOUR REVALIDATION JOURNEY

Early planning of the personal journey through revalidation will positively enhance the experience of the process. The ideal position is for registrants to have a written Personal Revalidation Plan as soon as possible. Using a well-structured plan, it will be possible for registrants to effectively deliver the requirements with as little stress as possible. As this is still a new process, there is still some anxiety about what to expect.

This chapter will provide information to support the development of a Personal Revalidation Plan. NMC registrants have sole responsibility for meeting the revalidation requirements. The NMC guidance (2015) states: "Revalidation is the responsibility of nurses and midwives themselves. You are the owner of your own revalidation process". During the development of the revalidation process, and subsequent to the launch, there has been much discussion about the role employers will play in the revalidation process. There is an emerging discourse among registrants that their career has now been placed in the powerful hands of employers, some of whom may not always prioritise the interests of registrants. This certainly can be the case, and is a theme to be addressed in the course of this book. It is possibly to revalidate efficiently with little or no support from employers, and this will be demonstrated throughout this book. Early planning is at the root of your ability to revalidate independently.

How to use support from employers

Registrants are recommended to view support employer support as an added extra to be incorporated into your Personal Revalidation Plan, rather than being that which their entire plan rests on. In this way, registrants will be in charge, but will be able to take account of any employer support as an added value. For some registrants, support from employers will be substantial and they will be able to meet all or most of the requirements through employer provision. However, it is very important to beware that changes in an employer's contribution will have to be accounted for in Personal Revalidation Plans, and contingencies will need to be put in place to reflect changes.

Changes may occur if a registrant changes jobs, if there are changes within an organisation, changes of line manager, or changes to a role within the organisation that may affect the support an employer is able to provide. These changes may result in loss of access to the support relied on to meet the requirements as part of registrants' employment. Most NHS and independent health care organisations are experiencing extreme financial pressures, and running deficits with the requirement to meet savings projections each year. Non-essential spending is being cut year upon year, and employers are under pressure to continuously identify savings. Savings plans have to be reviewed each year and support for NMC revalidation that an employer has been able to provide in the past may not be provided in future years.

Three Year Personal Revalidation Plan

The NMC recommends approaching revalidation on a continuous rolling basis, so that once successfully revalidated, registrants should then continue on with the range of activities that will allow them to meet the requirements for the next revalidation cycle. If registrants hold in mind that they are continuously ensuring they live the standards set out in the Code, documenting evidence in a portfolio over time, this will drive the development of Personal Revalidation Plans, as well as maintain focus on the purpose of revalidation – to protect the public and improve professional standards. Avoid taking the view that the purpose of revalidation is to tick off the minimum requirements, then sit back and not bring it to mind until it's time to prepare for the next revalidation application. The NMC recommends using the final 12 months prior to revalidation to arrange confirmation discussion meetings, once met all other requirements have been.

Start by developing a Three Year Personal Revalidation Plan which takes account of any other support such as that from employers or others. However, support, advice and assistance from your employer should not be the core element of the plan, as that is contingent on your employment with a particular employer, or being employed at all when you need to submit your revalidation application.

There are a number of steps to be followed to complete the process and scheduling these will be beneficial. Registrants will plan and schedule the steps in the process according to their own individual circumstances, however the following stages can be used as a guide:

Step 1: Take stock of the whole process and determine your support needs. This can only be achieved by reading through the current information on the NMC revalidation microsite as a starting point. Once read and understood, your working environment will guide your understanding of your support needs. Most NHS organisations have put arrangements in place to support their employees, and if you work for one of these you may find a lot of support available. This is very variable however. If you work outside the NHS, or on a self-employed basis, you will need to give careful planning and consideration to your overall support needs.

Most registrants have now registered with NMC Online, the portal that supports the electronic application. Once registered with NMC Online, you will be able to check your renewal date and when your revalidation is due.

Step 2: Liaise with the two key staff that will be essential to your revalidation application – your reflective practice discussion partner, and your confirmer. These can be the same person if NMC registered with a current effective registration. At an early stage book in your meeting with your reflective discussion partner, and then your confirmer, leaving a period of around a month between each meeting. This will allow you time to finalise your portfolio to provide the required assurance to your confirmer.

Step 3: Develop your portfolio, gathering all the evidence requirements, and completing the templates provided.

Step 4: Attend your reflective practice discussion meeting.

Step 5: Submit your online application form via NMC Online.

3 PRACTICE HOURS

Registrants must complete a minimum number of practice hours during the three year period since the last renewal or the period since first joining the register.

If you have more than one nursing registration, you still only need to complete a minimum of 450 practice hours to meet the requirement.

The requirements for compliance are clearly set out by the NMC's resources, therefore this chapter will focus on exploring solutions to potential issues. Chapter 8 on revalidating in diverse settings provides registrants with some issues and solutions on revalidation in diverse settings, and additional issues are considered here.

Issues
Evidencing practice hours for those diverse settings and scopes of practice.

Registrants who have worked continuously in one role, for a single employer over the three-year period prior to renewal, will find meeting this requirement to be a straightforward exercise. During the development of the NMC revalidation process, and prior to the publication of the final guidance, there was some concern about how registrants not working in direct patient care would meet the practice hours requirement.

This has now been clarified and those hours where a

registrant relies on their knowledge, skills and experience of being a registered nurse or midwife will count. The scope of practice (or field of work in which you practiced as a registrant), includes roles such as management, policy, commissioning, public health as well as direct patient care.

This is even if they are in roles which does not have a nursing or midwifery qualification as an essential requirement for the delivery of the role. A number of examples are provided here:
Example 1 – Housing Manager in the charity sector

A registered learning disability nurse who works as a housing manager in a residential facility for people with learning disabilities is likely to be able to use their hours in this role to meet this requirement. Their duties include assessing applications from prospective residents, assisting in the development of a resident's supportive living plan, recruiting, managing, supporting, and training a team of staff to meet the needs of the residents.

In this example, the manager is relying on her training, knowledge and skills as a learning disability nurse to do her day to day role in running the home. As long as the housing manager had a live registration during the course of working in her role, she is likely to be able to use those hours to meet the practice requirement.

Example 2 – Commissioning manager
A registered midwife currently working as a children and maternity commissioning manager in a Clinical Commissioning Group. This registrant therefore works in a diverse scope of practice but in a mainstream setting. On a day to day basis, she manages a portfolio of providers to ensure services are delivered in line with contract specification.

This includes running engagement and consultation exercises, listening to the views and experience of people who use the services, and using it to develop further commissioning plans or redesigning services. The registrant also work closely with clinicians, midwives and nurses to hear their views of services, how they are used, and how they can be improved. The commissioning manager's job specification does not include an NMC registration, but it is clear that she relies on the knowledge, skills, and experience as a registrant to deliver her role. As long as she had a live registration while working as a commissioning manager, she is likely to be able to use these hours to meet the requirement.

Example 3 – Trade Union Official
A trade union official is employed by a trade union representing health employees. The union official is a registered mental health nurse, and works closely with nurses, as well as other employees, advising on employment and practice compliance issues, and works as a caseworker supporting nurse and others in employment disputes. They also provide employee relations advise to employers, evaluate policies, and contribute to organisational service redesign and development. The union official was not required to be a registered nurse, however relies on her experience, knowledge and skills as a registrant to perform her duties. She has always maintained a live NMC registration, so is likely to be able to use these hours to meet the requirement.

Practice hours in diverse settings
Registrants employed in traditional settings such as hospitals, community services, and GP practices, Schools, Clinical Commissioning Groups, large social enterprises, and community interest companies will largely find meeting the practice hours requirement more straightforward than those in diverse settings.

Diverse settings are those where registrants now work but perhaps did not do so traditionally such as those employed directly by, for example, social care organisation, prisons, and in education. It also includes those who are self-employed, those working in agencies, and those directly employed by an individual. Action to meet the practice hours requirement The NMC has made arrangements for those in exceptional circumstances, for example those due to maternity leave, who are unable to meet the practice hours requirement. They will still need to meet the PREP standards, and are advised to contact the NMC well in advance of their revalidation date.

If a registrant does not meet the exceptional circumstances criteria of the NMC, action must be taken to complete the practice hours requirement. Undertaking regular voluntary or additional paid work as a registrant, will mean that you are likely to meet this requirement. Local health services, in the statutory and charity sector, can be approached. The additional practice hours can be for a different scope as long as you remain a registrant, and you rely on your skills, knowledge and experience to deliver the role.

Example 4
A part time mental health nurse works in direct patient care but his Personal Revalidation Plan show that he needed to top up his practice hours by 45 hours over three years. He volunteered to deliver 6 training days, over three years, in his own time, to a local children's mental health charity. This enabled him to top up the required practice hours, and contribute to his CPD, reflective practice, and practice-related feedback requirements

4 CONTINUING PROFESSIONAL DEVELOPMENT

Overview of NMC requirements:
- Undertake a minimum of 35 hours of CPD over the three-year period since last renewal/ revalidation
- Ensure 20 of the 35 hours are participatory learning
- Declare in your online revalidation application that you have met the CPD requirement.

In addition to this, you are recommended to maintain an accurate record of your of the CPD activities you undertook over the three years. You can do this in an e-portfolio or a paper-based portfolio. The NMC website contains a free template and worked example of their Continuing Professional Development Log Template which is recommended for use.

Registrants will be required to record the following:
- Dates you undertook the CPD

- CPD method (e.g. webinar, meeting, course or personal study)
- The topic studied
- How the topic is linked to the Code
- The number of hours/participatory hours

The CPD activity will only count if it is related to your scope of practice. As an example, if you are a dementia nurse, then a CPD activity on peer breastfeeding advisor programme may be of interest to you, but it will probably be queried if you include it in your CPD hours for revalidation purposes. Mandatory and statutory training will not ordinarily count

unless it is directly related to your scope of practice.
What counts as an appropriate CPD activity?
The NMC guidance, and worked examples on the NMC website gives some good suggestions, however it is left up to the registrant to decide what is an appropriate CPD activity. It is possible to meet the CPD requirement without any out of pocket costs to registrants or employers. The cost will be in the form of course the time taken spent in undertaking the activity, and that can may have an impact on an employer. If registrants will be undertaking CPD activities in their own time, this may have a number of impacts, particularly if they are attending classroom based learning activities.

Registrants who are employed by an employer that has a well –functioning appraisal scheme, should be able to undertake CPD as part of that scheme. However, many health service employers do not have effective appraisal schemes, and where they do exist, there may be other priorities that mean some registrants may not complete a full appraisal cycle in a timely manner. Many may experience an appraisal process that starts, but is not followed through with completion of paper work, or updates during the year. The next CPD cycle then starts, probably with a new line manager, which is based on an incorrectly completed, or incomplete previous appraisal cycle. As the NMC places responsibility for meeting the requirements with registrants, they should take ownership for their own CPD activities to meet the minimum requirement, even if it means using their own personal time. Ultimately registrants will need to decide the value of their registration.
Suggestions for CPD activities: Free non-participatory and participatory CPD

1. Library resources, books, national newspapers, and journals, library research events, online materials from almost any relevant source. Good resources include health websites such as NICE (The National Institute for Health and Care Excellence) which produces clinical evidence and guidance

for health and social care. Also try the websites of the Care Quality Commission (CQC), NHS Choices, Rethink the mental health charity, Midwifery Matters, The Practicing Midwife, The Royal College of Nursing and the Royal College of Midwives.

If you can obtain access to Athens database, this will give free access to a huge library of journal resources. Access to a health library at work should also will provide an Athens login, plus a wealth of resources. Those that don't work for an employer with such a resource, but live or work near one, then telephone the health library of your local NHS trust to find out if access for reference purposes only is available. Many health libraries are very under used, particularly by NMC registrants, and there may be scope to use the one at a local NHS trust through a negotiated agreement. Those who are self-employed, and develop a professional network locally, try asking a local health library to provide access for members of the network. If no access a specialist health library is available, local public libraries also have substantial health resources in book and journal formats. Local universities may also permit access to use their libraries by local people, and even if access is only for reference use, it would be beneficial.

2. Free talks and events

University talks and presentations, NHS Trust CPD sessions, breakfast meetings may be open not only to Trust staff, but other local professionals may be able to join, particularly if they contribute a talk. Many universities hold free talks and presentations open to the public, and on topics relevant to registrants, and as advance programme is available on their websites.

3. Exchange Visits and shadowing opportunities

This can be achieved by going to a meeting, it can be a regular meeting that you normally attend, where a relevant CPD opportunity can be undertaken if a relevant agenda item is presented. The meeting can be followed up by supplementary reading around the topic afterwards to develop a useful CPD activity. For example, an agency registrant working on a shift takes part in a 30-minute talk on mental health and diabetes. They took some brief notes during the session. The following week, on your day off, they went to their local library and did some online searches and found some useful journal articles on mental health and diabetes, and spent 2 hours reading them. This CPD activity counts as 2.5 hours, with half an hour as participatory.

4. Webinars
A lot of online learning now include webinars and if there is an opportunity for interaction, or to ask questions, and listening to the views, experiences or perspectives of others, they will count as participatory.

5. E-Learning for Healthcare
E-learning courses will count towards your CPD hours, but they are not usually participatory as an independent learner works through the structured programme. If learners decide to meet to discuss and perhaps amplify an aspect of the course, then that discussion meeting will count as participatory learning. An excellent, free online learning healthcare resource is e-learning for healthcare: http://www.elfh.org.uk/ and covers many short courses.

6. Public meetings of Trust Boards, Governing Bodies and Local Authority (also useful for reflective accounts)
This CPD activity is free of upfront costs and all geographic areas present these opportunities. Public sector organisations have a statutory duty to involve members of the public in a number of ways, and many of the events are highly relevant to the scope of practice for registrants. NHS Trusts, Social Enterprises proving health services, Clinical Commissioning Groups are required to hold part of their Trust Board or Governing Body meetings in public.

There is also an opportunity for members of the public to ask questions. Local Authorities also hold many of their meetings in public and the topics are again very relevant to registrants. The duty to involve also means there are often open public engagement and consultation meetings on topics relevant for registrants, and the sessions often include presentations and discussions. HealthWatch England has local groups that also act as the consumer voice for health, and often hold public events and consultation meetings, with presentations, sometimes for a whole day, that is very useful to attend. Community and voluntary sector groups often also hold engagement, and open days for local people, and focus on building community resilience and there are often presentations by health professionals on topics for the general public.

Low cost non-participatory and participatory • Voluntary and community sector training This training is intended primarily for the voluntary sector, and often includes topics relevant to registrants, and are often low cost, and sometimes even free.

5 PRACTICE-RELATED FEEDBACK AND REFLECTIVE ACCOUNTS

Overview of NMC requirements:
1. Obtain 5 pieces of practice related feedback during the three years since last renewal
2. Obtain feedback from a range of sources
3. Make a note of the feedback
4. Describe how you used the feedback to improve your practice

Practice-related feedback

The purpose of this requirement is to ensure nurses and midwives are taking every opportunity to be responsive to the needs of those they care for, their relatives and carers.

Feedback on care and treatment is given to nurses and midwives continuously by people who receive the care. Likewise, responding to this feedback is also a daily part of what registrants do as care professionals. However, there is evidence that there are gaps in the extent to which they sometimes respond to what patients tell us about their experience, and this requirement is intended to improve the performance of registrants and improve outcomes for people. Patient experience has been an essential part of quality in care services, and has increased in currency right across the health service in the past 10 years. There has always been interest in 'patient satisfaction' but that was skewed towards finding out what made patients happy, and with less focus on what makes patients unhappy, and what we can do to change that. The inquiry into the experience of patients at Mid Staffordshire NHS Foundation Trust between 2005 and 2009 was the critical recognition that staff failed to respond to the feedback of patients and carers. Nowadays, obtaining feedback from patients, expectant parents, and their friends and family is part of care that is provided. Registrants will be made aware of practice-related feedback from a range of sources. The NMC has made it clear that the feedback obtained by registrants do not all need to be about their own individual practice but can be about their service, team, or organisation.

Practice-related feedback can also be obtained from complaints, compliments, feedback in committee meetings, handovers, public consultation and engagement events, on websites or social media. There is a template available that the NMC recommends for use to record feedback, and is available on its revalidation microsite. As such, any suitable template will suffice, providing it only uses non-identifiable data. It must make no direct reference to an actual person, whether living or dead, or whether patient, service user or professional.

Reflective accounts
Overview of NMC requirements:
• Write a minimum of 5 reflective accounts over 3 years
• Write about CPD, Practice –related feedback or your professional practice and how it relates to the Code
 • A mandatory NMC recording form must be used
 • Discuss these reflective accounts with an NMC registered reflective discussion partner
• Confidentiality and data protection requirements must be maintained

Reflection is a core part of practice for nurses and midwives and they do it on a daily basis. Sometimes reflective practice in their daily work is structured and planned, at other times it is informal, snatched, instinctive and emergent. They also write reflections on a regular basis. Each time they write up patient notes, a care plan, or progress reports they are writing reflective accounts. Their records and notes include factual clinical information, and our perspective on the situation based on our own prior experience, professional training, and other factors.

All registrants will have experience of writing reflective accounts as part of initial training, CPD, or in post-graduate practice. However, many may not have consciously thought about written reflective accounts for some time, so it is refreshing to know how easy it is to harness what is done on a daily basis and turn it into the something that meets the NMC revalidation requirements.

Registrants can use this revalidation requirement as an opportunity to revisit or update their academic knowledge on reflective practice. That can then also feed into the CPD requirements. There are many opportunities to obtain up to date information on books, research articles on reflective practice. The NMC has strived to ensure that nurses and midwives are empowered as much as possible in this process, so there is a lot of scope for autonomy in how they approach writing reflective practice accounts, so this section is provided for support and guidance. The NMC has provided some examples of completed reflective practice accounts, and this chapter provides two additional examples.

Reflective account example One - Midwifery CPD example: What was the nature of the CPD activity and/or practice-related feedback and/or event or experience in your practice? This reflective account is about a CPD activity I undertook. The Information Services Division (Scotland), published a report in October 2015. This is a report about breast feeding statistics in Scotland during 2014 – 2015 and was published on the website of the Royal College of Midwives. I am a member of the Royal College of Midwives so received this information as an email alert.

What did you learn from the CPD activity and/or feedback and/or event or experience in your practice? I learnt that this study showed that the rate of breastfeeding has been largely unchanged in the last 10 years.

The most important and worrying part of the research is the difference in breast feeding pattern between the least and most deprived mothers, as the latter were three times less likely to breast feed than the former. As a midwife working in a deprived area of Scotland, our team was aware of this issue and frequently reviewed opportunities to make a positive impact and improve outcomes for the mothers and babies. We already have a number of initiatives and actions in place to improve access to breastfeeding for all mothers.

My main reflection on reading this report is problems that both my team, and I as an individual midwife have in assessing the deprivation levels of expectant mothers and how to address this in a sensitive way. We are also trained to treat all mothers equally, and not provide any with treatment and care that is seen as doing more' for some than others. However, this report and reflection opportunity increased my awareness that taking special measures to support deprived mothers will help them to access breast feeding support, advice and information to achieve the same outcomes as less deprived mothers.

There is also part of me that feels embarrassed, as someone who would fit into the category as 'less deprived', about acknowledging a new mother as ' more deprived'. It seems rude and impolite, and I would rather treat everyone the same, although on reflection that is not always the best approach. I suspect that some of the other midwives in my team might have similar feelings and this probably has an effect on our practice in providing deprived women with breastfeeding support.

How did you change or improve your practice as a result? Our service has a Midwifery Clinical Governance half day three times a year, and I decided that I would ask for this to be on the agenda for team discussion. I presented the report's findings at the next meeting, and asked the team to brainstorm some ideas on more actions or steps we could take to support more deprived women with breastfeeding. Of all of the ideas suggested we agreed on a focus group lunch event for mothers who had used the service and to discuss with them the needs of deprived mothers to enable us to learn from them.

How is this relevant to the Code? Select one or more themes: Prioritise people – Practice effectively – Preserve safety – Promote professionalism and trust.

This reflective account is relevant to the Prioritise people theme, particularly the requirement to "avoid making assumptions and recognise diversity and individual choice" and "respect the level to which people receiving care want to be involved in decisions about their own health, wellbeing and care". This reflection allowed me to see that while I feel comfortable in treating all women equally, and providing individual and personalised care, I needed to consider how to provide targeted and information, advice and support to women who are less deprived.

This reflective account is also relevant to the practice effectively theme in the NMC Code, particularly the requirement to "gather and reflect on feedback from a variety of sources, using it to improve your practice and performance" and to " maintain the knowledge and skills you need for safe and effective practice".
By presenting the paper, and leading the discussion in the midwifery clinical governance meeting, I was able to meet this theme and improve my effective practice.

Reflective account Two – CPD example at a Care Home
What was the nature of the CPD activity and/or practice-related feedback and/or event or experience in your practice? The relative of a resident gave me some feedback about one of our patients, Mr A, whilst I was on shift as the registered nurse for the home. The relative asked to speak with me at the end of her visit, and she was not happy with loud pop music being played on the lounge radio all the time. Her view was that as most of the residents were in later life, they may appreciate music they recognised rather than contemporary music which she said seemed to be played for the entertainment of the staff. I apologised for this situation, and said I would discuss it with the staff and the home manager and let her know what action we would be taking.

What did you learn from the CPD activity and/or feedback and/or event or experience in your practice? As most of the residents in the home had dementia and short term memory problems, it was unlikely that they would be very familiar with new pop songs, and I agreed with the feedback from the relative. This feedback was not new, and it had been raised before by visitors and family members. The home manager had talked to the staff about it, and they had made sure that appropriate radio stations were selected for playing in the resident's lounge.

How did you change or improve your practice as a result? As a registered nurse in the home I decided to raise it with the manager of the home, and agreed that I would also raise it at each handover over the coming weeks and ensure it was shared at each handover. I also brought in an article for all staff to read about respecting the needs of residents and maintaining their dignity.

How is this relevant to the Code? Select one or more themes: Prioritise people – Practise effectively – Preserve safety –

Promote professionalism and trust
I decided the practice effectively theme was most relevant to this feedback.

6 REFLECTIVE DISCUSSION AND CONFIRMATION

NMC reflective discussion requirements:
- You must have a reflective discussion with another NMC registrant about the five written reflective accounts you have completed.
- You must complete the approved NMC reflective discussion form and ensure it is signed by the reflective discussion partner.

Considerations registrants may wish to think about when developing a Personal Revalidation Plan are as follows:
Reflective discussion meetings and clinical discussions Consider how you might incorporate reflective discussions into your routine one to one sessions. In nursing and midwifery, the use of one to one sessions vary widely. At one end of the continuum, some sessions are used as a space for the allocation of work from line manager to supervisee, with the latter updating the former on progress.

At the other end, they are used as spaces entirely for supporting the supervisee with the space being used for them to gain support, and encouragement.

Revalidation for nurses and midwives reflect on their work. Some registrants have one to one sessions that are for clinical supervision, i.e purely for reflection on clinical work, as well as management supervision sessions which deals with HR matters, appraisal, and performance management issues. This is the usual arrangement in mental health nursing. In this scenario, it would make sense to use the cases discussed in clinical supervision for your reflective accounts, signing off the reflective discussion form after you have discussed the five cases you wish to use as evidence for your revalidation. You would need to follow the NMC's guidance to ensure no personal identification information is used in relation to any patient or professional.

Reflective discussion and group supervision
It is usual practice from some registrants, particularly in mental health care, to engage in group reflective discussion. There are different models however a typical approach is for a group of nurses, operating according to confidentiality rules within a team or organisation, meets regularly with each bringing a patient case for discussion and reflection. Each person discusses a case, and any management issues, actions they took, how they feel about the case, and obtain suggestions and support going forward. The group can be peer facilitated or can have a senior, advanced facilitator.

In the case of registrants, and nurses in the example given, this can be an opportunity to organically complete the NMC requirement on reflective discussion, provided the facilitator is a registrant, agrees to the process, and all rules on confidentiality and non-disclosure of any identifiable information relating to patients or professionals is adhered to. The NMC mandatory reflective accounts form can be completed prior to the session and each participant in the supervision session can discuss their cases as usual.

The NMC does not indicate exclusion of group-based reflective discussion, and in many cases as this will mirror what registrants are already doing, it is authentic, economical, meaningful and goes beyond a tick box exercise. Registrants are recommended to independently seek confirmation from the NMC to verify the use of local systems already in place to support their revalidation application.

One to one reflective discussion meeting
An approach that can be explored is that prior to reflective discussion meeting, the registrant sends their five reflective accounts to the discussion partner in advance. The reflective discussion partner can then review the reflective accounts and confirm whether they are able to proceed with the meeting or if the reflective accounts are not likely to meet the NMC requirements and needs further revision.

The registrant can then choose to undertake a review of their reflective accounts to ensure they meet the NMC requirement, and re-submit them to the discussion partner for review. If there is disagreement between the two at this stage, that cannot be resolved, it may be better for the registrant to seek a different discussion partner or seek advice from another registrant or their line manager.

If both are happy to proceed with the reflective discussion meeting, it is likely to proceed more smoothly. Registrants are free to structure the reflective discussion session as required, and the NMC provides a separate guidance sheet and presentation covering the essential requirements. Registrants will be very pressed for time, however they should agree well in advance of the meeting, the time to be taken, as well as the structure and format of their reflective discussion.

If all five reflective accounts are to be discussed in one sitting, it is wise to allow a minimum of one and a half hours, although two hours is more realistic, particularly for complex scopes of practice.

Aim to agree in advance whether the meeting will be completely informal and unstructured, or whether there will be an agenda. Some registrants will be having reflective discussions with partners they do not know, and possibly have never met, and this will guide the advance decision making about structure and format of the meetings. An outline agenda could be structured in the following way:

Agenda
1. Introductions (5 minutes)
2. Presentation of the first account. Registrant reads through reflective account from the form. (5 minutes)
3. Discussion partner asks questions, discusses account, and seeks clarification (5 minutes) These two stages are repeated until all reflective accounts have been discussed
4. Discussion partner asks any residual questions about the five cases, and gives feedback to the registrant. (10 minutes)
5. The paperwork is signed by the discussion partner, who makes a copy for their own records, giving the original to the registrant. (5 minutes)
6. The registrant and discussion partner discuss the verification process and confirm whether the discussion partner agrees to be contacted by the NMC as part of the verification process and to cooperate with that process. (10 minutes)
7. Summarise and close

This agenda supports a meeting of one hour and 10 minutes, and provides only a brief time slots for discussion of the accounts. A meeting that genuinely allows time to reflect, and learn from this process will need more time.

Using alternative arrangements for reflective discussion meeting

The NMC suggests that a face-to-face meeting is the ideal way of conducting a reflective discussion meeting, and failing that, a video conference could be arranged.

Many registrants will not have access to video conferencing arrangements as these are normally reserved for executive or senior staff within NHS organisations, however, if they are available, they are a good alternative to a face to face meeting. Registrants may also wish to consider using Skype which they can do at home or work if the facilities are available.

Telephone conference calling may also be a suitable alternative, but less preferable as there is no face to face contact and non-verbal communication is very important for effective overall communication.

No complex equipment is required as most modern telephones have a speaker facility, which will allow hands-free two-way telephone call. If a third party is to be involved in the reflective discussion, they can be involved in the meeting in this way also.

Confirmation - Overview of NMC requirements
• Obtain confirmation from an appropriate confirmer
• Make a declaration that you have demonstrated your compliance with the regulations to an appropriate confirmer
• Use the NMC mandatory form to record the confirmer's details, and sign off of the process

This part of the revalidation process may require significant involvement from non-registrants and the NMC has produced a separate guidance document for confirmers. This role is so critical to a registrants career it has come under particular scrutiny, and discussion. The NMC has emphasised its belief that:

'Your line manager is an appropriate confirmer, and we strongly recommend that you obtain confirmation from your line manager wherever possible. A line manager does not have to be an NMC-registered nurse or midwife.'

Registrants are further advised to seek out an NMC registered confirmer in the first instance, but if one is not available, to ask another regulated professional such as a doctor, dentist, or pharmacist. An online confirmation tool is available on the NMC website that assists registrants to identify other possible confirmers. This tool will lead registrants to further lists of potential confirmers.

First level confirmer– NMC registered Line Manager Second level confirmer – Non NMC registered Line Manager

Third level confirmers:
Art therapist
- Biomedical scientist
- Chiropodist
- Chiropractor
- Clinical scientist
- Dentist
- Doctor
- Dietician
- Hearing aid dispenser
- Occupational therapist
- Operating department practitioner
- Optician
- Optometrist
- Orthodontist
- Orthoptist
- Osteopath
- Paramedic
- Pharmacist
- Physiotherapist
- Psychologist
- Podiatrist
- Prosthetist / orthoptist
- Radiographer
- Social worker
- Speech and language therapist

Fourth level confirmers:
Accountant (with professional qualifications)
- Acupuncturist (with professional qualifications)
- Barrister
- Chemist

- Commissioner of Oaths
- Engineer (with professional qualifications)
- Fire Service Official
- Judge
- Justice of the Peace
- Lawyer
- Legal Secretary (members and fellows of the Institute of Legal Secretaries)
- Member of Parliament
- Merchant Navy Officer
- Minister of a recognised religion
- Officer of the armed services (active or retired)
- Police Officer
- Registration Authority/Licensing Board
- Solicitor
- Surveyor (with professional qualifications)
- Teacher / Lecturer (with professional qualifications)
- Veterinarian
- Ward manager

So there registrants will clearly not run out of options for people who will be able to confirm their application. So with this wide range of potential confirmers, what are the main issues for confirmation process?

1. Honesty and integrity

There are a number of reasons why a confirmer may fail to act honestly and in good faith when tasked with undertaking the role. These reasons may be personal; such as conflict with the person the confirmer is acting for. Because a person is in a senior role does not mean they will act in an honest, and professional manner. The risk is that such a confirmer will act with malice and fail to confirm a registrant's evidence, requiring them to unnecessarily resubmit aspects of the evidence, causing delay that then causes the registrant to miss their application deadline and result in a lapsed registration.

Line Managers may have priorities that conflict with their role as a confirmer, and result in them not completing the confirmation in with honesty and in good faith. This applies to NMC and non-NMC registrants, and other regulated health professionals. The NMC has a priority on recommending confirmers who are regulated, in the hope that they are more likely to act with integrity and good faith, but above all the can be held to account for breaches of their professional code should they act dishonestly.

2. Lack of understanding by employers of the revalidation process Employers may inadvertently conflate the revalidation process with the requirements of their employment of the registrant. They may incorrectly decline to confirm the registrant, and can act to prevent other employees to act as confirmer for a registrant on the basis of an employment issue.

The NMC has stated that: "Revalidation is not an assessment of a nurse or midwife's fitness to practise, a new way to raise fitness to practise concerns or an assessment against the requirements of their current or former employment" (Employer's Guide to Revalidation, NMC, 2015) The strands of this statement will be quite complex for some employers to detangle, as many will not be familiar with existing NMC regulation. Training and education on the new NMC revalidation has been mainly targeted at registrants, and whilst this will be cascaded to employers, and others, time will be needed for full understanding to be obtained by all employers. In the meantime, registrants need to take responsibility for ensuring misunderstandings and misinterpretations by employers of the revalidation process does not adversely impact them.

Third level confirmers

These are regulated health professionals that often work closely or in partnership with nurses and midwives. They may not have prior experience of playing such a critical role in the regulation of NMC registrants and their involvement requires careful organisation and planning. They are all busy professionals and to undertake the role and deliver it effectively, accurately they will need to commit many hours. They will need to read and understand the NMC guidance for confirmers, and may want to read the full range of guidance documents on the website for registrants to optimise their understanding of the requirement.

In addition, it is important that they have a pre-meeting with the revalidating registrant. Holding a pre-meeting between registrant and confirmer is strongly recommended by this book for all confirmations, however if two NMC registrants are confident about the process, have received training on NMC revalidation, it is not essential. However, for a third level confirmer, who wishes to support registrants in with revalidation, a pre-meeting will assure both parties that they are on the same page.

Should it be a mandatory requirement that third level confirmers attend a training session before they undertake confirmation? It is advisable. Reading the guidance documentation is unlikely to be sufficient to meet the needs of those who have no prior experience of NMC regulatory processes. A further consideration for NMC registrants in seeking confirmation from a third level confirmer is to consider how this might change the dynamics of the relationship between nurses and midwives, and their professional colleagues who now have a role in their regulation.

There may be no change, or there may be a change if problems occur and there is a challenge to the evidence provided by the confirmer who has possibly not understood their role, or the evidence.

Thought will also need to be given to what would motivate a third level confirmer to want to add hours to their workload? Time will be needed to read materials, possibly attend training session, have a pre-meeting, and then a confirmation meeting, as well as making themselves available thereafter for the verification process.

NMC registrants have great partnerships and alliances with third level confirmers, however there may need to be a motivating factor, to obtain support from third level confirmers. There could possibly a benefit to their own CPD or professional portfolios as an incentive. There may be an anxiety for regulated health professionals that they might be putting their own registration or professional status at risk by acting as an NMC confirmer. In the event they inadvertently provide information that subsequently turns out to be incorrect, the NMC has made it clear it will not take action against confirmers in these circumstances. Attendance at training sessions on the requirements of NMC revalidation will help to reduce these anxieties and provide third level confirmers with the information they need.

Fourth level confirmers

Most of the issues outlined for third level confirmers are relevant to fourth level confirmers. There is less scope, however, for these confirmers to have easy access to training about the role, except for ward managers. They also have less or no experience of working with NMC registrants and may have a limited understanding of NMC regulation. To ensure effective confirmation by fourth level confirmers, a pre-meeting is strongly recommended, and the registrant is advised to assure themselves that their confirmer has all the information required.

Choosing a confirmer

According to the NMC guidance, registrants are at liberty to choose their own confirmer, however the close alignment between NMC revalidation and employer processes, such as line management confirmation, and employer appraisal schemes may reduce how much choice registrants have. Registrants may find themselves in the position of having their confirmer allocated to them, or of being informed that their line manager is the only person who will act as confirmer.

However the guidance states registrants have a right to choose, and if a line manager is imposed as confirmer, registrants are advised to query this, unless fully satisfied with this arrangement. It is advisable to choose very carefully, and avoid choosing a confirmer if you believe there is a chance that they may not act in good faith.

Whist you may be able to subsequently complain or initiate action against an NMC registrant, or other regulated professionals who fails to act in good faith and deliberately cause a lapsed registration, it is best to act to avoid it. Only choose a confirmer that you are completely confident about. It is best to avoid a problem than seek to correct it later, as it will be a very costly consequence.

Some registrants will make the decision early on that their line manager is not someone they will choose to act as confirmer, and they will need to inform them of this, and be aware that this may cause problems if they were expecting to act as confirmer.

You can justify this if you are part of a professional network that has agreed to support each other with reflective discussions and confirmations on a reciprocal basis.

Some registrants may prefer to use independent confirmer, a registrant outside their employment and professional networks. Some scenarios featuring issues that may affect registrants seeking confirmation is presented here. It also looks at how independent confirmers, can be used as part of the process.

Example 1
A midwife has been working for an employer for 6 months, and raised concerns due about standards in the service during this time. This has caused tension between her and her line manager and the latter has declined to act as confirmer, and other midwives in the team have said they are unable to act as her reflective discussion partner. The midwife has 6 months left to revalidation, and her reflective discussion and confirmation meetings are still outstanding.

What can you do if you find yourself in this situation?
There are a number of issues for the registrant, however the clear priority is to independently make arrangements for a reflective discussion partner and confirmer. The registrant has the option of using registrants from her previous employment, or professional networks that she may be part of. However, if neither of these options are possible, and if she has trade union membership, that may be another source of help. Consider external, including professional paid-for revalidation services as an option once assured yourself of the quality of the service.

Example 2
A registrant is subject to formal sickness absence management procedures by her employer, and is at Stage 2. She is currently at the start of a 6 month monitoring plan. She is due to submit her revalidation application soon and has her confirmation meeting still outstanding. Her line manager

has declined to complete the confirmation stage pending the completion of the sickness absence monitoring process. No fitness to practice issues have been raised.

What can you do if you find yourself in this situation? This registrant is entitled to proceed with her revalidation process, however the employer cannot be required to support her. The priority is to secure a reflective discussion partner, and a confirmer as soon as possible, from the range of options discussed in Example 1.

Tips for all registrants
Make arrangements early and keep them under review, as it can be difficult to find an appropriate confirmer with short timescales. Registrants approaching prospective reflective discussion partners and confirmers very late notice may give rise to concerns about their practice and questions about why their employer has declined to provide support, and they may also decline. The registrants in both examples may want to consider using paid-for revalidation services, but they must assure themselves that there is no conflict of interest in the way the services are provided. Paid for educational, training, coaching services are already provided to registrants on a professional basis without compromising the integrity of the service. It is also in the registrant's interest to satisfy themselves that any paid-for services are undertaken with honesty and integrity. These examples can be used to indicate that conflict of interest issues are not necessarily a risk only from paid-for revalidation services:

Scenario 1
A group of nurse registrants working on the same ward start to make arrangements to act as reflective discussion partners and confirmers. They are a close team of best friends who also socialise regularly and go on holiday together. Registrant A is not completely confident that Registrant B that she has been paired with has met all the requirements, but registrant

B has already signed off the forms for registrant A. Registrant A decides to sign off the documentation anyway. At the point of verification, the NMC notifies Registrant B that her registration is at risk because of the quality of evidence provided in her portfolio. In this scenario, a conflict of interest has arisen due to the close friendship that exists in the teams.

Scenario 2
Re-read the midwifery registrant scenario in this chapter. Having exhausted all of her options, she engages the services of an NMC registrant, a part time midwifery lecturer, who also provides revalidation services on both a free and paid for basis, depending on the amount of input required. She reviews the registrant's situation, and agrees to offer a reflective discussion meeting and a confirmation meeting, provided in a single session, at the same Band 7 hourly rates as her substantive practice. She agrees to charge only for the face to face hours, and to review the paperwork in her own time. The services are provided to a high standard and the midwife is successfully revalidated. She is selected for the NMC revalidation process, and no issues are raised and her revalidation is fully verified. All registrants will need to be aware that registrants cannot charge another registrant for confirmation services.

Registrants will need to be aware that for confirmation meetings as with reflective discussions, pre-planning is important, including advance forwarding of the paperwork to the confirmer.

Confirmation meetings with multiple parties Some registrants will want their confirmation meetings to be attended by more than one confirmer. If they work part time and have two line managers, they may wish them both to be present, but with one leading on the confirmation. Some registrants may have a mentor, or professional adviser they wish to invite. This approach may be particularly relevant where a confirmer is not a health professional. Further, in the first year of NMC revalidation, it is useful to provide others with the opportunity to shadow the confirmation process, particularly where they are third or fourth line confirmers.

This could also be the solution where a line manager has been imposed, and the registrant wishes to have a third party present. This meeting is so critical to a registrants' future career, that over time, it may come to be viewed as too critical to be left to the judgement of a single confirmer.

Agenda
The confirmation meeting is naturally more structured than reflective discussion meetings, as the NMC provides a clear checklist of what the confirmer needs to see and do. However, an agenda will assist with budgeting the time available, and keeping the meeting on track. A sample agenda is provided as follows:

Confirmation meeting Agenda
1. Introductions (5 minutes)
2. Practice hours requirement – Practice hours log template presented by registrant (10 minutes)
3. Continuing Professional Development – CPD Log template presented by registrant (10 minutes)
4. Five pieces of practice related feedback – written or oral evidence presented by registrant (15 minutes)
5. Five written reflective accounts – written accounts presented by registrant (15 minutes)
6. Reflective discussion – a completed and signed NMC form recording that the registrant has held a reflective discussion with an MNC registered nurse or midwife (5 minutes)
7. Discussion of any issues, agreement on whether the mandatory requirements have been met (10 minutes)
8. Signing of confirmation form by confirmer (5 minutes)
9. Discussion of verification, and agreement that the

confirmer will be available to participate in the verification process if the registrant is selected for verification.

Alternatives to face to face meetings As with reflective discussion meetings, it is possible to make other arrangements such as video conferencing or conference calling if a face to face meeting is not possible.

7 APPLICATION AND VERIFICATION

Important: The revalidation application deadline is the First Day of the month in which your registration expires

Application Registrants can submit their online application to the NMC from 60 days prior to renewal, when their online application portal will open. It is advisable to submit the application and complete the revalidation in plenty of time before the renewal date. Be aware that you will also need to pay your renewal fee before the registration is renewed for a further three-year period. Once your revalidation application has been successful, your registration will be renewed from the date it is due to expire. Registrants will need to set up an NMC Online account before being able to apply for revalidation.

This can be done through the NMC website, and will enable registrants to check their renewal date. The NMC has made provision for those who need reasonable adjustments to be made to allow them to submit their applications. This is in line with the Equality Act (2010) and includes those who are native Welsh speakers who trained in the Welsh language. Once you are ready to start your online application, you are advised to ensure you have all the evidence and documents you need to hand.

This includes your paper portfolio, or e-portfolio. Registrants will be notified by email from the NMC on the outcome of their application. If your application is found to have failed to meet the requirements, your registration will lapse and you will no longer be able to practise as a nurse or midwife. To re-join the register, you will need to apply to the NMC for readmission, and meet the revalidation requirements. There is a process of appeal against an NMC decision to reject a revalidation application.

Those who require the following considerations should contact the NMC:
1. Reasonable adjustments for using NMC Online
2. Exceptional circumstances claims
3. Extension requests

Registrants need to be aware of the serious implications of a lapsed registration, due to recent changes meaning there is no longer an administrative window from November 2015. Those registrants who fail to renew their registration will immediately be taken off the register. This is in keeping with promoting professionalism, and self-responsibility which is consistent with NMC revalidation.

Verification
The NMC will select a sample of registrants to request further evidence and information from, and they will be notified immediately on submitting their application, or within 24 hours. If selected, they will need to complete an online form, and possibly also asked to provide evidence that they have met the revalidation requirements as declared.

They will need to alert their confirmer, reflective discussion partner, and employer that they may be contacted by the NMC for more information. If a confirmer or reflective discussion partner fails to respond, this will jeopardise your revalidation application. This is another reason to exercise great care in the choice of reflective discussion partner and confirmer, and ensure you are confident they will respond if subsequently contacted by the NMC for verification purposes.

8 REVALIDATION IN DIVERSE SETTINGS AND SCOPES OF PRACTICE

Registrants work in very diverse settings and scope of practice, and the NMC aimed to reflect this during the pilot phase of the revalidation process. This chapter looks at the issues for registrants working in nursing homes, for agencies, GP practices, and those who are self-employed. It also includes registrants in diverse scopes of practice that does not involve direct patient care.

Meeting the requirements in diverse settings

IT Access

IT access is taken for granted by those working for large organisations, however it is not always available to registrants working in diverse settings. There are registrants who have no computer access at work, and have no computer at home. This includes not having an email address and no access to the internet. Options in these cases involve registrants having to make use of the free computer and internet access available in some public libraries, and internet cafes. This is very limiting, and can be costly over a period of time. Registrants who will be completing NMC revalidation are strongly recommended to purchase a computer (desktop or laptop), and good used models are available with warranties. To access the internet, options are to purchase an internet service to use at home, or to purchase mobile internet service in the form of a 'dongle' from any high street mobile phone provider. Having your own computer and internet service at home will hugely improve the revalidation experience for you and may reduce costs of using external computer and internet services overall. Networks, for example of independent or self-employed registrants can consider purchasing a laptop for the network that can then be loaned within the network. In theory, the only part of the process that requires a mandatory online process for NMC revalidation is the revalidation application which must be made via NMC Online. Registrants will therefore need to ensure they have organised IT access well in advance of the 60-day period leading up to the deadline for renewal.

Bank and Agency nurses and midwives
Challenges and Solutions Registrants who work on a short term, temporary, locum basis will need to plan carefully to ensure they are able to meet the requirements of the new NMC revalidation scheme. Bank workers are those who are recruited directly by organisations such as NHS Trusts, to work on a flexible, ad hoc basis.

They are a very cost effective resource, and usually highly valued. They can find themselves working in a number of different settings to meet the staffing levels of the organisation, but can also find that they mostly work in the same ward or other setting for extended periods.

Agency or locum workers are those placed in healthcare settings, to complete an assignment, normally a single shift. They are directly recruited and employed by organisations who run their own trust bank or sometimes even an internal agency. Temporary workers are faced with a number of challenges that can all be overcome, and solutions found, if careful and early planning is put in place.
1)   Meeting the practice hours requirement.
 This is the same as for arrangements under PREP, so is not a new challenge. What temporary workers do need to ensure is that they are able to evidence that they meet the hours. They will need to retain timesheets and other records of hours worked. As timesheets are mainly weekly this could result in

registrants having to store large quantities of paper. The suggested tip here is to work with your bank or agency to obtain quarterly, six-monthly or annual statements of the hours worked. An alternative is for employers or agencies to produce certificates of hours worked, again on a quarterly, six-monthly or annual basis. These are simple steps that employers and agencies can take to make an otherwise burdensome aspect of the requirement more streamlined. Temporary workers who are self-employed may choose to keep all timesheets for tax purposes, but it will still be more convenient for portfolio development to have a summarised sheet of hours worked.

2) Continuing Professional Development requirement. Most temporary registrants will only be supported by their agencies or employers to access statutory and mandatory training. The first strategy here is to talk to your employers to see what additional support they can provide to enable you to meet the requirements. This may simply be supporting the setting up of professional networks among registrants, or identifying a scheme to put people in touch with each other. Provision of learning resources, and access to IT learning facilities would be of great support to its staff. Agencies are in a great position to negotiate with NHS trusts that they regularly provide staff for, to enable them to access in-house training, or library facilities.

3) Professional indemnity cover requirement. If you work in the NHS through an agency with an NHS contract , or through its bank, you should check if you are covered by the Trust indemnity scheme, which is the usual arrangement. You will need to obtain evidence of this for your portfolio, and NHS Trusts will be able to provide this for you. Again, this is something agencies can support you with. As NHS organisations will need to provide this for all their NMC registrants, over time, it can be expected that a simple system will be developed to make this available. Agency registrants

who do not work in the NHS may find they are covered by the service they work in, such as with an independent organisation. Those who provide services in an individual's home, for example, will need to investigate the cover they will need.

4) Reflective accounts, feedback, reflective discussion and confirmation requirements. Agency and bank workers working in the NHS will have similar opportunities to substantive staff to write reflective accounts, access practice-related feedback, find a reflective discussion partner and a confirmer. However, this will vary widely between organisations and some temporary workers will find they are not able to access this support from their employer. External agencies may have to request revalidation support for their staff, particularly those that work regularly for the organisation. As an alternative, external agencies will need to develop their own support schemes. They can develop a database of their own registrants who are prepared to act as reflective discussion partners or confirmers. They can also provide resources such as office space on their premises that can be used for meetings.

GP practices

Practice nursing teams vary in number, but many practice nurses will have good access to other nurses. The challenges and solutions share some similarities with bank and agency registrants. Many registrants working in GP practices will be able to meet the practice hours requirement, and will not have significant issues evidencing how they have met it. Continuing Professional Development requirement: GP practice registrants will largely be supported by their employers to maintain their competencies through CPD. Those that do not receive this support are advised to take two options. Firstly, set out a support scheme to present to employers, mapped against the numbers of registrants employed. Secondly, take steps to set up a professional network with registrants in local practices.

Such networks can take time to set up, and will require employer support, and much advance planning. They can also be challenging to set up, and general advice is provided later in this chapter. However, for the setting up of professional networks between practices, this is one example of an approach that can be followed:

a) Project Leadership: Identify two or three people from different practices to lead the network project. Approach the setting up of the network as a managed project. This will ensure the load is shared, and there is buy in from more than one practice.

b) Plan: The project leadership should plan the objectives, roles and resources needed, and implementation of the network, focusing on a developing a long term plan, of at least 1 year.

c) Make it professional. Agree terms of reference, agenda, meeting spaces, meeting frequency, agenda, and agree to rotate who will be responsible for taking and distributing minutes. Revalidation is about promoting professionalism among registrants, so it makes sense to take a professional approach to setting up and running a network.

d) Keep it simple: an approach would be monthly meetings for all members, for two hours. Members take turns to present topics, or invite external speakers. Attendance will always be an issue, so for practices an evening network may be preferable.

e) Broaden membership: the network will be richer if the membership is broadened to include registrants outside of those working in local practices, that is part of the decision making for the project leadership group. Membership could be opened to all registrants in the region, or area, such as town or city.

f) Funding: the project team can hold early discussions with the membership to identify if there will be a membership fee. The benefits are that it will strengthen commitment and attendance if an annual membership fee is paid for in advance. A membership fee will also provide funds for resources such as meeting rooms, and fund events such as workshops, conferences, and pay for external speakers.

g) Specialise: registrants can choose to establish a professionals network around a specialist clinical topic of interest to members. All meetings can be centred on this topic, and be for members specialising in that topic only.

h) Time limited networks: networks may wish to establish only for set time periods, to allow time to evaluate, review, and establish new networks in response to emergent needs and contexts. For example, GPs are currently commissioning leaders in their local region and that has an impact on general practices. If this changes in the future, practice nursing teams may wish to re-configure to take account of changes. Further, NMC revalidation progresses, learning will guide the development of the network, and the initial period can be treated as a pilot phase. i) The issues that may affect nurses working in GP practices in relation to reflection discussion and confirmation meetings, can be addressed by the discussion points in chapter 6.

Nursing homes
1. Challenges and Solutions
Nurses working in care homes will also have a varied experience, but it is common to be provided with a good amount of employer support for CPD to enable this requirement to be met. The solutions to reflective discussion and confirmation challenges can be met through reviewing

the section for those working in GP practices as they will also work well with care home practitioners.

2. Self- employed registrants
Nurses and midwives working on a self- employed basis are likely to need to take specific action, and early planning to ensure they meet the requirements. The practice hours requirement: this has not changed from the PREP requirements, so self- employed registrants will already have processes in place to meet this, however chapter 3 also provides information and suggestions.

Continuing Professional Development: self-employed registrants will already be responsible for arranging their own CPD activities and may have strategies in place. However, chapter 4 suggests a number of approaches that may be useful for self-employed practitioners. 35 hours CPD is almost a working week in terms of hours, which can be costly for self-employed practitioners Reflective discussions and confirmation meetings for self-employed practitioners means networking is essential, either through other contacts you meet in the course of your work, or through the setting up, or joining of local, regional or national networks.

Membership of a trade union or professional body will also assist with connecting with other registrants who can act as reflective discussion partners, and confirmers if needed. Professional indemnity: self-employed registrants will need to take advice to ensure they are covered as this is a complex area. Most will already have this in hand as a requirement of provide services on a self-employed basis.

Some self-employed registrants may be covered by the NHS if they provide services to the NHS, but this need to be confirmed. There are many sources of indemnity cover such as trade unions, professional bodies, and general insurance providers and once covered, the evidence should be retained in a portfolio for verification purposes.

Meeting the requirements in diverse scopes of practice
Registrants working in education, policy, commissioning, transformation, project and programme management, and service management who wish to maintain their registrations much revalidate. This also includes nurses and midwives who rely on their skills, knowledge, and experience of being a registered nurse or midwife, but are in roles where their employment contract does not expressly require them to be registered with us. For example, this could include roles in public health or nursing or midwifery management, commissioning, policy and education. See chapter 3 for discussion of the challenges and solutions for those working in diverse scopes of practice.

Networks and networking
The NMC has stated that one of the reasons why it introduced revalidation for nurses and midwives is "to encourage you to engage in professional networks and discussions about your practice".

The value of professional networks is undeniable both for NMC registrants, their patients and the public that benefits from their expertise. Whilst there are many networks available for nurses and midwives to participate in, many would argue that the reality is that most do not engage with networks for a number of reasons.

The main reason is lack of time for NMC registrants to be released from direct patient care settings to attend network meetings. A second key reason is lack of employer support to be provided with on-site meeting spaces for network meetings to be held. For registrants who are not directly employed, or working for agencies or on a bank basis, the problems of networking are even more concentrated. Finally, there is an administrative and organisational burden in running a network, and there may be a requirement for IT access which is not available to all NMC registrants.

Despite these barriers, many registrants work in settings where they will have good opportunities to network with other nurses and midwives, and can collaborate together, and with employers, to put good local revalidation schemes in place. Barriers to setting up and running good networks can be overcome or managed, particularly if they are operated external to employers. Networking is necessary for sharing information, getting support, and getting help with the critical reflective discussion and confirmation requirements of revalidation.

For example, most employers will probably look favourably on a nursing and midwifery revalidation network or scheme run within the organisation. Some employers will support and even fund networks with schemes in place to ensure equitable access for all registrants to support in meeting the NMC requirements.

If formal schemes are not put in place, nurses and midwives will rely on informal friendship networks, which might leave some out in the cold, lead to resentment, anxiety and inequality.

Some registrants may find themselves oversubscribed with requests to act as reflective discussion partners, or confirmers which may impact on their time management and planning. Similarly some nurses and midwives will play a minimal role in providing this support to others.

To avoid these pitfalls, revalidation networks can establish schemes that deliver the following:
• Annual forward mapping of NMC registrants, and all renewal dates on an annual basis
 • Have a rolling monthly programme of information and

briefing sessions for registrants
• Develop a programme of face to face CPD sessions free to participants
• Support planned access to reflective discussion partners and confirmers

Types of networks
1. Face to face networks – registrants will already be part of a number of specialist networks for nursing and midwifery, where they have regular contact with others working in a similar field. They will usually be attending in their capacity as a service provider or other practitioner in policy, commissioning, education etc. The purpose of these networks is to discuss a fixed agenda, however issues of professional practice do emerge and sometimes can be the focus of the discussion. These networks can be good launch pads for setting up professional practice networks where registrants meet with an agenda purely on practice.

2. Online networks are increasing in popularity (see chapter 9 on social media) and are often linked to physical events, or Meetups, which are a great way to bring people together for learning and developing. Some online networks remain virtual, with members only interacting online, which also has significant professional value, particularly for those in diverse settings and scopes of work who might not have the opportunity to meet with others or join in debates outside of this these networks.

9 SOCIAL MEDIA AND REVALIDATION

This chapter explores how registrants can use social media (SoMe) to support their portfolio development and meet the revalidation requirements. It also to introduces registrants to the some of the main SoMe platforms. SoMe is no longer an optional tool for health services, as its use is now almost universal in healthcare in the UK. Before participating in SoMe as a registrant, nurses and midwives are advised to review the NMC guidance document Guidance on Using Social Media Responsibly. The key point made in this guidance is that registrants using social media must remember they are still bound by the standards set out in the NMC Code (NMC, 2015). Registrants are asked to hold three standards in mind to guide their conduct on social media sites and platforms:

1. Be Informed – educate yourself about different social media, know how they work and their potential value and the risks of using them.

2. Think Before You Post – Be aware of the limitations of privacy settings on anything you post as it can probably be made publicly available.

3. Protect Your Professionalism and your reputation – Be aware your reputation may be inadvertently compromised through the online action of your social media associates.
Technology in general, and SoMe specifically is developing at a such rapid pace that it is difficult to keep abreast of developments, and identify benefits for healthcare.

However, to ignore SoMe as a healthcare professional is to place yourself at a significant disadvantage, and risk losing a multitude of learning and development opportunities, many of which will be useful in meeting the NMC revalidation requirements.

This chapter will look at five popular SoMe platforms, and provide a brief overview of how they can be used as tools to help you meet the NMC revalidation requirements. People are also ambivalent about using SoMe in the workplace as we are just now moving away from the position where employers blocked staff access to these sites, and barred their use in the workplace, regarding them suspiciously as only having leisure, recreational and personal value.

A residual impact of this is that staff in some organisations still feel as if they are breaking rules if they use SoMe sites for work reasons, during work time. However, most employers now have a presence on SoMe sites, and these accounts are normally operated by communications departments as a key interface between the organisation and the public. Some individuals who never contact health organisations directly or visit their websites do use social media, and it is a great way of interacting with a different range of patients and members of the public.

Common features of SoMe:
• Cyberbullying is a feature of SoMe when abuse is directed towards organisations for individuals. Trolling is a form of cyberbullying where a user deliberately posts content with the sole intention of starting a n argument or causing offence, and typically targets individuals.
• Spamming is the use of computer generated accounts to target SoMe users, often for commercial purposes, selling products, but also for the circulation of malware and viruses. The standard rule applies is make sure you are certain of the sender of any content before you engage with it.

- Spamming can also occur if your account is taken over and used to send out spam contents to your followers or friends. This is managed through the regular changing of your passwords, and not leaving your account dormant as those are the most at risk of takeover by spammers.

- Blocking is a feature common to most SoMe introduced to give users some protection against cyberbullying and spamming. These are features that allow you to block another user from viewing your site or interacting with you any further.

- Campaigning is now an integral part of SoMe and registrants may at some point be approached to sign an online petition.

- Meetups are increasingly popular offshoots of connections made online, where participants will meet informally, or in a structured way for workshops or conferences linked to the subject that brought them together online.

- You will need to make a decision about whether your SoMe account is personal or professional, and this is a very grey area. Most employed professionals clearly indicate on their accounts whether it is professional, or whether they are running the accounts in a personal capacity. If the latter, they often have a disclaimer that the account does not reflect the views of their employer but are purely personal.

With NMC registrants, care is needed as the Code states "You uphold the reputation of your profession at all times" so it is best to bear this in mind on SoMe.

Blogging

A blog is defined and operated in various ways. Most commonly, it is an online personal diary or journal of content provided by an individual. The term blog is used interchangeably for both the website used to host the blogs, and the individual entries made by the author. A blog can also be any website such as a subject website operated by one or more individuals on various topics, with contributions from many others.

The term blog is also used to refer to an article contributed to a website that is not a blog, for example an NHS Trust can feature the CEO's monthly blog. The common theme in blogging is the sharing of reflections on a topic. Blogs can be a rich source of information about the experience of patients and service users as many write blogs about their experience of treatment for a range of conditions including mental health conditions, and physical health conditions, and their experience of using specific services.

Facebook
Facebook is a social network with hugely flexible uses for health services. Once an account is opened, users can set up a page that is then used to share information about their organisations, including events, developments, and for recruitment. It can be used as a way for the public to make contact with the organisation to provide comment, and feedback based on their experience of using the services.

Content can be pictorial, audio visual, or narrative announcements. Many NHS and non-NHS health services have Facebook accounts and they use them on a regular basis to provide updates about the organisation. It is a rich source of feedback, information and interaction between patients and the public. As well as organisations, teams or individual practitioners and services also set up accounts or pages, and share content, and receive feedback from patients and members of the public. Privacy controls are available, but this is less likely to be an issue for organisations and health professionals who are using SoMe in order to reach larger audiences.

Twitter

Twitter is a micro-blogging SoMe platform. It is a social networking site where users can publish tiny 'blogs', or phrases, up to 140 characters, providing content such as updates, pictures, audio-visual, and video streaming from other SoMe sites. To 'tweet' is to post content using a twitter account, and because of the brevity of the content, and the rapid sharing of information by millions of users, there is a lot of 'noise', with the tweets appearing as rapid bursts of content. To 're-tweet' is to redistribute, or share someone else's tweet with your followers. This is normally interpreted as an endorsement of the original tweet, and even though you may include a disclaimer in your profile about re-tweets, you are still sharing someone else's tweet, which equates to tweeting.

As with Facebook, most NHS and many non-NHS healthcare organisations, teams, services and health professionals now have twitter accounts.

The key features of twitter is the use of the 'hashtag', which is now prevalent across a lot of social media. A hashtag is the use of the symbol # before a word, without a space, which will cause it to be aggregated with all other tweets that use the same hashtag. People interested in that topic can then view all the tweets on that subject. So #revalidation or #NMCrevalidation are examples of hashtags than can be viewed on twitter.

Webchats or tweetchats are hosted structured discussions organised on twitter for interested participants. The date and time, and host are arranged in advance. The host can be the same person as the chair or facilitator but there can be a host and a chair for some chats. Formats are varied and emerging but they all centre around the use of an appropriate hashtag to ensure everyone is linked in and can see all the contributions of the other speakers.

They normally last for an hour, and the conversations can be summarised and shared by using other SoMe tools such as Storify, which pulls together all of the contributions in a single document which is then shared with all participants for later reflection, and discussion as required. Trending is also a key feature of SoMe sites, most commonly associated with twitter. Trending is when a topic, usually with a hashtag but not always, is used with very high frequency on twitter. So during a Webchats, if a hashtag is used by a large number of participants in a short period of time, it 'trends' and is listed in a topic list of the highest trending topics.

Top Twitter Accounts to follow for NMC revalidation:
1. @nmcnews (The Nursing and Midwifery Council)
2. @KaterinaKolyva (Dr Katerina Kolyva, NMC)
3. @WeNurses; @WeMidwives; @WeMHNurses
4. @joan_myers OBE (Joan Myers)
5. @theRCN (The Royal College of Nursing)
6. @YvonneCoghill1 & @RogerKline (NHS England Workforce Race Equality)
7. @Nursingtimesed (JenniMiddleton)
8. @AgencyNurse (Teresa Chinn MBE RN)
9. @JaneMCummings (Jane Cummings) 10. @NM_revalidationhelp

YouTube

YouTube is a video sharing social media site. It is used by many health professionals, services and organisations to share filmed content about their services for patients, and members of the public. Typical content shared is corporate organisational information, but also content about patients and service users speaking about their experience of using services, and providing feedback for prospective users. Health Boards now also post videos of their board meetings, for example NHS England, and the Care Quality Commission are all online to view. Other examples of content on YouTube useful to registrants include the NSPCC, MacMillan Cancer, NMC Safeguarding Adults, Statutory Safeguarding Children's guidance, mental health trusts, Clinical Commissioning Groups, Midwifery and Practice nursing. Viewers of the content have some opportunity to comment but this is restricted.

Periscope

Periscope is owned and operated as part of Twitter. It is a live broadcasting SoMe platform where users can broadcast live. Health professionals are using Periscope to broadcast live feeds of events, conferences, talks, and meetings. They also host Q&As about health topics and give talks themselves. Combined with presentations, this is a low cost way of sharing and learning.

A smartphone is necessary to use Periscope which is available as an app. Once you have set up an account, you follow other users that you follow on twitter, plus others, and you also acquire followers. You then receive notifications if any of the people you are following has started a live broadcast which you can join. Your followers similarly receive notifications of your broadcasts which can be watched live or as a replay. The advantage of watching live is that you get the opportunity to interact through text communications with the broadcaster who then responds verbally to your communications.

Broadcasts are stored for 24 hours on Periscope, but can also be saved in a permanent form. Registrants are recommended to explore opportunities to use SoMe to assist them in portfolio development, and in meeting the NMC revalidation requirements. There are opportunities to learn how to use SoMe with online tutorials, particularly on YouTube.

10 LESSONS LEARNED SO FAR

Several months into the new revalidation process, many lessons have been learned by those who have gone through the process, and those supporting others. This chapter sets out and discusses the commonly reported experiences of registrants and those obtained from my experience of supporting registrants through the process.

The experience of registrants going through the process is extremely variable, as predicted, because of the diverse circumstances and settings in which they work. Registrants working within the same setting, and even within the same work area have been reporting very different experiences. These differences do lie with individual approaches to revalidation, but it is also dependent upon the level of support provided within the setting.

Employer support
The ideal circumstance that contributes to a successful and positive experience of revalidation is where registrants are line managed by other registrants who are informed and positive about revalidation. Such managers provide team briefings on revalidation where team members of all disciplines are made aware of the process and that they have a part to play in supporting members who are registrants. These managers are proactive and aware of the revalidation dates and support requirements of all registrants in their team.
The opposite scenario is where a registrant is line managed by

a registrant who is not an NMC registrant and is not informed or interested in the process. It is certainly true that some managers who are registrants are not informed or positive about the process, but as they are fellow registrants they are required to take an interest in the subject because they will also be required to go through the process, unless they intent to let their registration lapse before their renewal is due. In this situation, registrants can find themselves struggling to get through the process alone and having to find support outside of their team or work setting.

Emotional experience
This is mixed and depends on support provided, and individual approach. A sense of panic, worry and anxiety is still widespread, particularly among registrants who have undertaken little preparation of the process. Those who have taken the time to become fully informed of the requirements tend to feel more in control, and less anxious. They are reporting the experience as simple, straight forward, enjoyable and empowering and enjoy celebrating successfully revalidating with colleagues.

They are reporting a real sense of achievement. The most enjoyable part of the process appears to the reflective accounts, and the reflective discussion. Registrants are saying they appreciated this and are don't often, or not at all, get the opportunity to discuss and reflect in detail on their nursing practice. Supervision for nurses, where it happens at all, is often focused on management topics, with little consideration given to in-depth discussion of practice. Some registrants are saying that this is the first time they have had such a discussion since they qualified indicating that reflection is seen as useful during the training period, but not in qualified practice.

Organisation and planning
This is also individual with a mixture of approaches being taken. Although many registrants are taking at least minor steps in the process, it is only when they receive the letter or email from the NMC two months in advance of their renewal date that many really become focused. Some start the process only after receiving this notification. A minority are still in the position of not knowing their revalidation date not having acted on the notifications from the NMC, resulting in lapsed registrations. There is still a 'head in the sand' approach where registrants are in denial that they have to go through this.

Registrants with a positive and organised approach to revalidation, who have fully engaged with the process are tending to take a three year, cyclical view of the process.

Challenges
Several months into the process registrants have identified some common themes as challenging. Firstly, many have said they find the writing requirement difficult. They have found writing all elements of the requirements very difficult because they have not current experience of writing in this way. Many have not written for nursing practice for a long time, since they were last students. The challenge of writing the reflective accounts, the CPD learning benefits and writing about their reflections on feedback have all required a lot of effort. This has been a source of stress to registrants in the process. This is understandable as registrants are not required to write in this way in day to day practice and these skills have become rusty over a period of time.

When selecting practice-related feedback, two common issues have been observed. Firstly, most registrants are only selecting direct feedback from patients/service users/relatives and colleagues about them as individual practitioners. They are not making use of the wealth of feedback to the team or even organisation that provides great scope for learning and development. Secondly, most are providing positive feedback as examples, and I have yet to see any negative or mixed feedback. This is may be indicative of worry about being blamed or even reported if negative practice related feedback, particularly if personal. The potential for learning from negative practice-related feedback is very significant, however not all registrants feel they work in supportive environments, or with supportive managers who are skilled in listening to negative practice related feedback.

Registrants are able finding it problematic to find someone to act as reflective discussion partner or confirmer. Problems related to not having a line manager because of a vacant post where a manager has left and their post has not been recruited to. There may be another manager from another area who has been asked to cover that area on a temporary basis, as well as their own area. The function of the covering manager is not to cover all the tasks, and they tend to focus on managing the clinical function, shifts, and staffing levels and not much more.

Even when there is an appropriate line manager, registrants are hesitant in asking their manager to book in a reflective discussion and/or confirmation meeting. This is a confidence issue in some cases, particularly because they are asking their senior to undertake an additional task. They may not have a good relationship with their manager, and often this arrangement is vague, and not booked in, just a general undertaking that it will be done.

The experience to date as reported by those in diverse settings has also been very variable. Some registrants working for agencies or nurse banks have reported surprise at how supported they have been. Many have received all the support they need through their agency, or if working through a bank, have found that they have been treated as members of the team if working on long term assignments.

As anticipated, colleagues in the private nursing home and primary care sectors are finding they require more planning and thought to identify processes to ensure they revalidate successfully.

Finally, there were many fears about an online process, and the experience to date is that those registrants who were already comfortable with IT have found the process smoothest. Those who do not use the internet, and there are many employed registrants who work for NHS trusts who never or rarely use the internet, have found it a great challenge. They have relied heavily on others, including colleagues, friends, family, and even their young children, to assist them with the IT aspect of their revalidation.

References and resources
Chief Nursing Officer Letter (October 2015) https://www.gov.uk/government/uploads/system/uploads/attachment_data/file/477757/CNO_Nurses_Midwives_Revalidation_Letter.pdf
SENGE, P. M. (1990). The fifth discipline: the art and practice of the learning organization. New York, Doubleday/Currency. MID STAFFORDSHIRE NHS FOUNDATION TRUST 2013. Report of the Mid Staffordshire NHS Foundation Trust Public Inquiry - Executive summary London: Crown Copyright.
NMC revalidation resources
http://www.nmc.org.uk/standards/revalidation/

ABOUT THE AUTHOR

Claudia Tomlinson is a registered mental health nurse successfully supporting registrants through the revalidation process since implementation in April 2016. She is a, psychology graduate, independent nurse prescriber, qualified teacher and experienced practitioner. She is also qualified NVQ assessor (Level 3 Certificate in Assessing Vocational Achievement) with substantial experience in coaching, training and mentoring.

Her current scope of practice is in a diverse setting, and she has worked in a range of settings including NHS Trusts, community, mental health, and commissioning and project management environments. Since April 2016, she has been providing support to registrants, acting as a reflective discussion partner and confirmer and successfully supported registrants to complete the revalidation process. She is also a blogger with the Independent Voices, and Huffington Post UK. She is active on social media platforms, and runs the blog:

Revalidation Help for Nurses and Midwives:
http://revalidationhelp.wix.com/nurse-revalidation

Printed in Great Britain
by Amazon